Copyright

While every Precaution has been taken in the preparation of this book, the Publisher assumes no responsibility for errors or omissions, or damages resulting from the use of the information contained herein.

Tired of Acne Skin?

Second Edition. November, 2019.

1

LEGAL DISCLAIMER

The information in this eBook is not intended to replace medical advice.

No action or inaction should be taken based solely on the contents of this information.

Before beginning this or any other nutritional or exercise regimen, consult your physician to be sure it is appropriate for you.

The information and opinions expressed here are believed to be accurate, based on the best judgement of this author.

Readers who fail to consult with appropriate health authorities assume the risk of any injuries.

ALL RIGHTS RESERVED.

Table of Contents

5

Acne an Overview

Acne is an inflammatory Problem of the skin caused by the clogging of hair follicles with oil and dead cells that often times leads to bacteria invasion.

Acne normally starts in forms of initial whiteheads/blackheads which later develops into pustules/papules and gradually become severe and leads to formation of scarring and cystic nodules.

Therefore early detection and accurate treatment of Acne is highly recommended to avert the worsen conditions. Acne normally appears like multiple pimples, bumps or painful red lumps on the face or any other parts of the body such as the neck, back and shoulder. This can be quite disturbing for teenagers and some adults especially when acne appears on the face. It will cause embarrassment and make one feel inferior to others.

Some People can be so worried and ashamed of the urgly look on their face and would not be able to face the crowd.

What exactly are the Causes of Acne?

The main causes of Acne are:

1. Excessive sebum (Skin oil) production.
2. Excess androgens.
3. Bacteria invasion of the skin.
4. Clogging of the hair follicles with sebum

Some home remedies can help to Prevent Acne

• Wash affected areas twice daily and gently.

• Avoid scrubbing affected areas when having your bath.

• Avoid using oily creams.

• Avoid cleansers with gritty contents.

• Reduce intake of chocolates and skimmed milk.

• Do not squeeze or use your hands to pick on Acne in order to prevent scar formation.

• Do not use astringents that will dry up the skin.

• Avoid prolonged intake of corticosteroids.

Drinking 6-8 glasses of water daily keeps the skin hydrated and toxin free.

Regular exercises daily keeps the skin pores open due to sweating and reduces the risk of acnes

Acne Treatment

Most acne usually responds to topical therapy though a combination of oral and topical therapy is more effective. Successful treatment depends mainly on the use of product that follows the below guide

1. Inhibition of sebum production
2. Limitation of bacteria growth
3. Promotion of shedding of cells to unclog skin pores.

There are 4 Major Factors to Consider When Choosing an Acne Product

1. The uses of natural products such as plant based supplements are more tolerable because they do not have side

11

effects unlike orthodox acne creams.

2. Choose a product that has a cream and capsule supplement to attack acne internally and externally.

3. Choose a product that can eliminates all forms of blackheads/whiteheads

4. Choose products that are highly rich in antioxidants such as vitamin C, E and Aloe-Vera to protect your skin from bacteria invasion.

Adult acne

The number of adults who have acne is growing.

Why treat acne?

Myths about acne are as common as the skin problem. One common myth is that you have to let acne run its course.

Dermatologists know that letting acne runs its course is not always the best advice.

Here's why:

Without treatment, dark spots and permanent scars can appear on the skin as acne clears.

Treating acne often boosts a person's self-esteem.

13

Many effective treatments are available.

More women getting acne

Not just teens have acne. A growing number of women have acne in their 30s, 40s, 50s, and beyond. Dermatologists are not sure why this is happening. But dermatologists understand that adult acne can be particularly frustrating.

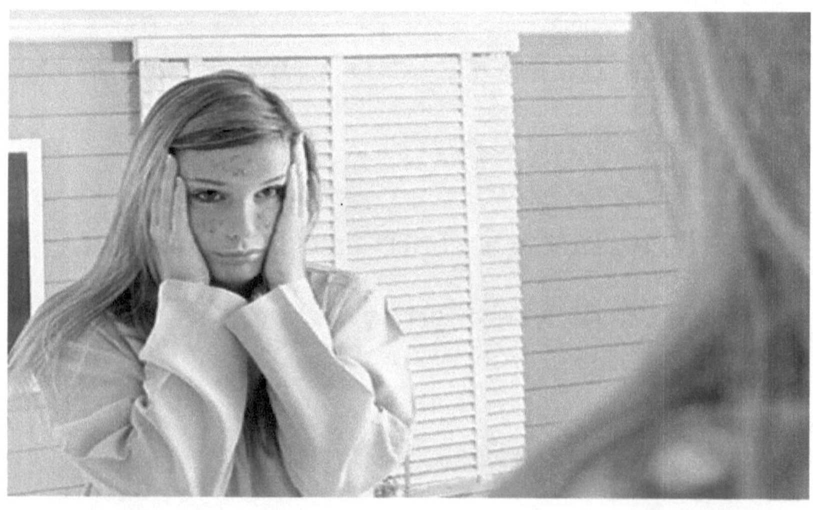

Acne: Signs and Symptoms

Acne signs

Many people think that acne is just pimples.

But a person who has acne can have any of these blemishes:

Blackheads

Whiteheads

Papules

Pustules (what many people call pimples)

Cysts

Nodules

Acne can appear on the back, chest, neck, shoulders, upper arms and buttocks.

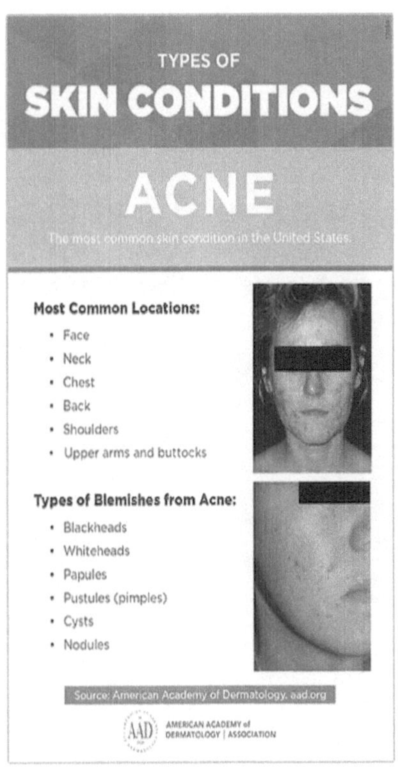

Acne symptoms

Acne can cause more than blemishes. Studies show that people who have acne can have:

Low self-esteem

Many people who have acne say that their acne makes them feel bad about themselves. Because of their acne, they do not want to be with friends. They miss school and work. Grades can slide, and absenteeism can become a problem because of their acne.

Depression

Many people who have acne suffer from more than low self-esteem. Acne can lead to a medical condition

18

called depression. The depression can be so bad that people think about what it would be like to commit suicide. Many studies have found that teens who believe that they have "bad" acne were likely to think about committing suicide.

Dark spots on the skin

These spots appear when the acne heals. It can take months or years for dark spots to disappear.

Scars (permanent)

People who get acne cysts and nodules often see scars when the acne clears. You can prevent these

19

scars. Be sure to see a dermatologist for treatment if you get acne early—between 8 and 12 years old. If someone in your family had acne cysts and nodules, you also should see a dermatologist if you get acne. Treating acne before cysts and nodules appear can prevent scars.

What you need to know about Acne.

Acne is a chronic, inflammatory skin condition that causes spots and pimples, especially on the face, shoulders, back, neck, chest, and upper arms.

Whiteheads, blackheads, pimples, cysts, and nodules are all types of acne.

It is the most common skin condition in the United States, affecting up to **50 million** Americans yearly.

It commonly occurs during **puberty**, when the sebaceous glands activate, but it can occur at any age. It is not dangerous, but it can leave skin scars.

The glands produce oil and are stimulated by male hormones produced by the adrenal glands in both males and females.

At least **85 percent** of people in the U.S. experience acne between the ages of 12 and 24 years.

Fast facts on Acne

Acne is a skin disease involving the oil glands at the base of hair follicles.

It affects 3 in every 4 people aged 11 to 30 years.

It is not dangerous, but it can leave skin scars.

Treatment depends on how severe and persistent it is.

Risk factors include genetics, the menstrual cycle, anxiety and stress, hot and humid climates, using oil-based makeup, and squeezing pimples.

Home remedies for Acne

Acne is a common skin problem.

23

There are many suggested home remedies for acne, but not all of them are supported by research.

Diet

It is unclear what role diet plays in worsening acne. Scientists have found that people who consume a diet that offers a good supply of vitamins A and E and of zinc may have a lower risk of severe acne. One review describes the link between acne and diet as "controversial," but suggests that a diet with a low glycemic load may help.

Tea-tree oil

Results of a study of 60 patients published in the *Indian Journal of Dermatology, Venereology, and Leprology* suggested that 5-percent tea-tree oil may help treat mild to moderate acne.

If you want to buy tea-tree oil, then there is an excellent selection online with thousands of customer reviews.

Tea

There is some evidence that polyphenols from tea, including green tea, applied in a topical preparation, may be beneficial in reducing sebum production and treating acne. However, the compounds in this case were extracted from tea, rather than using tea directly.

Moisturizers

These can soothe the skin, especially in people who are using acne treatment such as isotretinoin, say researchers. Moisturizers containing aloe Vera at a concentration of at least 10 percent or witch hazel can have a soothing

26

and possibly anti-inflammatory effect.

Causes

Human skin has pores that connect to oil glands under the skin. Follicles connect the glands to the pores. Follicles are small sacs that produce and secrete liquid.

The glands produce an oily liquid called sebum. Sebum carries dead skin cells through the follicles to the surface of the skin. A small hair grows through the follicle out of the skin.

Pimples grow when these follicles get blocked, and oil builds up under the skin.

Skin cells, sebum, and hair can clump together into a plug. This plug gets infected with bacteria, and swelling results. A pimple starts to develop when the plug begins to break down.

Propionibacterium acnes (P. acnes) is the name of the bacteria that live on the skin and contribute to the infection of pimples.

Research suggests that the severity and frequency of acne depend on the strain of bacteria. Not all acne bacteria trigger pimples. One strain helps to keep the skin pimple-free.

Hormonal factors

A range of factors triggers acne, but the main cause is thought to be a rise in androgen levels.

Androgen is a type of hormone, the levels of which rise when adolescence begins. In women, it gets converted into estrogen.

Rising androgen levels cause the oil glands under the skin to grow. The enlarged gland produces more sebum. Excessive sebum can break down cellular walls in the pores, causing bacteria to grow.

29

Other possible triggers

Some studies suggest that genetic factors may increase the risk.

Other causes include:

- Some medications that contain androgen and lithium
- Greasy cosmetics
- Hormonal changes
- Emotional stress
- Menstruation

Acne: Who Gets and Causes?

Who gets acne?

If you have a bad case of acne, you may feel like you are the only one. But many people have acne. It is the most common skin problem in the United States. About 40 to 50 million Americans have acne at any one time.

Most people who have acne are teenagers or young adults, but acne can occur at any age. Newborn babies can get acne. Men and women get acne. Some women get acne when they reach middle age.

What causes acne?

Acne appears when a pore in our skin clogs. This clog begins with

31

dead skin cells. Normally, dead skin cells rise to the surface of the pore, and the body sheds the cells. When the body starts to make lots of sebum (see-bum), oil that keeps our skin from drying out, the dead skin cells can stick together inside the pore. Instead of rising to the surface, the cells become trapped inside the pore.

Sometimes bacteria that live on our skin, *P. acnes*, also get inside the clogged pore. Inside the pore, the bacteria have a perfect environment for multiplying very quickly. With loads of bacteria inside, the pore becomes inflamed (red and swollen).

If the inflammation goes deep into the skin, an acne cyst or nodule appears.

Acne Diagnosis and Treatment

How do dermatologists diagnose acne?

To diagnose acne, a dermatologist will first examine your skin to make sure you have acne. Other skin conditions can look like acne. If you have acne, the dermatologist will:

Grade the acne. Grade 1 is mild acne. Grade 4 is severe acne.

Note what type, or types, of acne appear on your skin.

How do dermatologists treat acne?

Today, there are many effective acne treatments. This does not mean that every acne treatment works for everyone who has acne. But it does mean that virtually every case of acne can be controlled.

People who have mild acne have a few blemishes. They may have whiteheads, blackheads, papules, and/or pustules (aka pimples). Many people can treat mild acne with products that you can buy without a prescription. A product containing benzoyl peroxide or salicylic acid often clears the skin. This does not mean that the acne will clear overnight.

Despite the claims, acne treatment does not work overnight. At-home treatment requires four o eight weeks to see improvement. Once acne clears, you must continue to treat the skin to prevent breakouts.

When to see a dermatologist

If you have a lot of acne, cysts, or nodules, a medicine that you can buy without a prescription may not work. If you want to see clearer skin, you should see a

35

dermatologist. Dermatologists offer the following types of treatment:

Acne treatment that you apply to the skin

Most acne treatments are applied to the skin.

Your dermatologist may call this topical treatment.

There are many topical Acne treatments. Some topical help kill the bacteria. Others work on reducing the oil. The topical medicine may contain a retinoid, prescription-strength benzoyl peroxide, antibiotic, or even salicylic acid.

Your dermatologist will determine what you need.

How to Apply Topical Acne Medication

Today, there are many effective treatments for acne. To get the greatest benefit from topical acne medications, follow these tips from board-certified dermatologists.

Acne treatment that works throughout the body

Medicine that works throughout the body may be necessary when you have red, swollen types of acne.

This type of treatment is usually necessary to treat acne cysts and nodules.

Your dermatologist may prescribe one or more of these:

Antibiotic (helps to kill bacteria and reduce inflammation).

Birth control pills and other medicine that works on hormones (can be helpful for women).

<u>**Isotretinoin**</u>

Procedures That Treat Acne

Your dermatologist may treat your acne with a procedure that can be performed during an office visit.

These treatments include:

Lasers and other light therapies:

These devices reduce the *P. acnes* bacteria.

Your dermatologist can determine whether this type of treatment can be helpful.

Chemical peels:

You cannot buy the chemical peels that dermatologists use.

Dermatologists use chemical peels to treat two types of acne—blackheads and papules.

Acne removal: Your dermatologist may perform a procedure called "drainage and extraction" to remove a large acne cyst. This procedure helps when the cyst does not respond to medicine. It also helps ease the pain and the chance that the cyst will leave a scar.

If you absolutely have to get rid of a cyst quickly, your dermatologist may inject the cyst with medicine.

41

Possible Outcome

Waiting for acne to clear on its own can be frustrating. Without treatment, acne can cause permanent scars, low self-esteem, depression, and anxiety.

To avoid these possible outcomes, dermatologists recommend that people treat acne. When the skin clears, treatment should continue. Treatment prevents new breakouts. Your dermatologist can tell you when you no longer need to treat acne to prevent breakouts.

42

Acne: Tips for Managing.

HOW TO TREAT A DEEP, PAINFUL PIMPLE

Although acne comes in many forms, including blackheads and whiteheads, the most severe type of acne is a pimple that develops deep in the skin, causing a red, swollen, and painful bump.

To treat this type of pimple at home, follow these tips from dermatologists to alleviate pain and reduce the pimple's size, swelling, and redness.

43

You can reduce your acne by following these skin care tips from dermatologists.

Wash twice a day and after sweating.

Perspiration, especially when wearing a hat or helmet, can make acne worse, so wash your skin as soon as possible after sweating.

Use your fingertips to apply a gentle, non-abrasive cleanser.

Using a washcloth, mesh sponge, or anything else can irritate the skin.

Be gentle with your skin.

Use gentle products, such as those that are alcohol-free. Do not use products that irritate your skin, which may include astringents, toners and exfoliants. Dry, red skin makes acne appear worse.

Scrubbing your skin can make acne worse.
Avoid the temptation to scrub your skin.

Rinse your body with lukewarm water

Shampoo regularly.

If you have oily hair, shampoo daily.

Let your skin heal naturally. If you pick, pop or squeeze your acne, your

45

skin will take longer to clear and you increase the risk of getting acne scars.

Keep your hands off your face. Touching your skin throughout the day can cause flare-ups.

Stay out of the sun and tanning beds. Tanning damages you skin. In addition, some acne medications make the skin very sensitive to ultraviolet (UV) light, which you get from both the sun and indoor tanning devices.

Using tanning beds increases your risk for melanoma, the deadliest form of skin cancer, by 75%.

Consult a dermatologist if:

- Your acne makes you shy or embarrassed.

- The products you've tried have not worked.

- Your acne is leaving scars or darkening your skin.

- Today, virtually every case of acne can be successfully treated.

- Dermatologists can help treat existing acne, prevent new

47

breakouts and reduce your chance of developing scars.

- If you have questions or concerns about caring for your skin, you should make an appointment to see a dermatologist.

Acne Treatments

Treatment depends on how severe and persistent the acne is.

Mild acne

A variety of steroidal and non-steroidal creams and gels are available to treat acne, and many are effective.

Mild acne can be treated with over-the-counter (OTC) medications, such as gels, soaps, pads, creams, and lotions that are applied to the skin.

Creams and lotions are best for sensitive skin. Alcohol-based gels dry the skin and are better for oily skin.

OTC acne remedies may contain the following active ingredients:

Resorcinol: helps break down blackheads and whiteheads

49

Benzoyl peroxide: kills bacteria, accelerates the replacement of skin, and slows the production of sebum

Salicylic acid: assists the breakdown of blackheads and whiteheads and helps reduce <u>inflammation</u> and swelling

Sulfur: exactly how this works is unknown

Retin-A: helps unblock pores through cell turnover

Azelaic acid: strengthens cells that line the follicles, stops sebum eruptions, and reduces bacterial growth. There is cream for acne, but other forms are used for rosacea.

It is advisable to start with the lowest strengths, as some preparations can cause skin irritation, redness, or burning on first use.

These side effects normally subside after continued use. If not, see a doctor.

Treating moderate to severe acne

A skin specialist, or dermatologist, can treat more severe cases.

They may prescribe a gel or cream similar to OTC medications but stronger, or an oral or topical antibiotic.

Corticosteroid injection

If an acne cyst becomes severely inflamed, it may rupture. This can lead to scarring.

A specialist may treat an inflamed cyst by injecting a diluted corticosteroid.

This can help prevent scarring, reduce inflammation, and speed up healing. The cyst will break down within a few days.

Oral antibiotics

Oral antibiotics <u>may be</u> <u>prescribed</u> for up to 6 months for

patients with moderate to severe acne.

These aim to lower the population of *P. Acnes*.

The dosage will start high and reduce as the acne clears.

P. acnes can become resistant to the antibiotic in time, and another antibiotic is needed. Acne is more likely to become resistant to topical rather than oral antibiotics.

Antibiotics can combat the growth of bacteria and reduce inflammation.

Erythromycin and tetracycline are commonly prescribed for acne.

53

Oral contraceptives

Oral contraceptives can help control acne in women by suppressing the overactive gland. They are commonly used as long-term acne treatments.

These may not be suitable for women who:

- Have a blood-clotting disorder
- Smoke
- Have a history of <u>migraines</u>
- Are over 35 years old

It is important to check with a <u>gynecologist</u> first.

Topical antimicrobials

Topical antimicrobials also aim to reduce *P. acnes* in patients with moderate to severe acne. Examples are clindamycin and sodium sulfacetamide.

The dermatologist may prescribe a topical retinoid.

Topical retinoids are a derivative of vitamin A.

They unclog the pores and prevent whiteheads and blackheads from developing.

Examples of topical **retinoids** prescribed in the U.S. are

55

adapalene, tazarotene, and **tretinoin.**

Isotretinoin

This is a strong, oral retinoid, used for the treatment of **severe <u>cystic acne</u>** and severe acne that has not responded to other medications and treatments.

It is a strictly controlled medication with potentially serious side effects. The patient must sign a consent form to say that they understand the risks.

Adverse effects include dry skin, dry lips, nosebleeds, fetal abnormalities if used during pregnancy, and mood swings.

Patients who take isotretinoin must avoid vitamin A supplements, as these could lead to vitamin A toxicity.

Types of Acne and How to Treat Them

Acne types

You may hear the term **"breakout"** used to describe all forms of acne, but this isn't always an accurate description. Not all types of acne spread across the skin.

57

Clogged pores cause acne itself. These may be attributed to:

- excess production of oil (sebum)
- bacteria
- hormones
- dead skin cells
- ingrown hairs

Acne is usually associated with hormonal fluctuations experienced during your teenage years, but adults can experience acne, too. About **17 million Americans** have acne, making it one of the most common skin conditions among both children and adults.

Identifying which type of acne you're experiencing is key to successful treatment.

Acne may be **non inflammatory or inflammatory**. Subtypes of acne within these two categories include:

- blackheads
- whiteheads
- papules
- pustules
- nodules
- cysts

It's possible to have multiple types of acne at once — some cases may even be severe enough to warrant a visit to the dermatologist.

Non inflammatory acne

Non inflammatory acne includes blackheads and whiteheads. These normally don't cause swelling.

They also respond relatively well to over-the-counter (OTC) treatments.

Salicylic acid is often marketed for acne in general, but it usually works best on non inflammatory acne. It naturally exfoliates the skin, removing dead skin cells that can lead to blackheads and whiteheads.

 Look for it in cleansers, toners, and moisturizers.

Blackheads (**open comedones**)

Blackheads occur when a pore is clogged by a combination of sebum and dead skin cells. The top of the pore stays open, despite the rest of it being clogged. This results in the characteristic black color seen on the surface.

Whiteheads (**closed comedones**)

Whiteheads can also form when a pore gets clogged by sebum and dead skin cells.

But unlike with blackheads, the top of the pore closes up.

It looks like a small bump protruding from the skin.

Whiteheads are more difficult to treat because the pores are already closed. Products containing salicylic acid can be helpful. Topical retinoids give the best results for comedonal acne. Currently, adapalene (Differin) is available over the counter as a retinoid. If it does not work for you, stronger topical retinoids are available by prescription from your dermatologist.

Inflammatory acne

Pimples that are red and swollen are referred to as inflammatory acne.

Although sebum and dead skin cells contribute to inflammatory acne, bacteria can also play a role in clogging up pores. Bacteria can cause an infection deep beneath the skin's surface. This may result in painful acne spots that are hard to get rid of.

Products containing benzoyl-peroxide may help reduce swelling and get rid of bacteria within the skin. These can also remove excess sebum. Your doctor may prescribe either an oral or topical antibiotic along with the benzoyl-peroxide to treat your inflammatory acne.

Topical retionoids are also an important part of combatting inflammatory papules and pustules.

Papules

Papules occur when the walls surrounding your pores break down from severe inflammation. This results in hard, clogged pores that are tender to the touch. The skin around these pores is usually pink.

Pustules

Pustules can also form when the walls around your pores break down. Unlike papules, pustules are filled with pus. These bumps come out from the skin and are usually red in color. They often have yellow or white heads on top.

Nodules

Nodules occur when clogged, swollen pores endure further irritation and grow larger. Unlike pustules and papules, nodules are deeper underneath the skin.

Because nodules are so deep within the skin, you can't typically treat them at home. Prescription

65

medication is necessary to help clear these up.

Your doctor or dermatologist will likely prescribe the oral medication isotretinoin (Sotret). This is made from a form of vitamin A and is taken daily for four to six months. It can treat and prevent nodules by decreasing oil gland size within the pores.

Cysts

Cysts can develop when pores are clogged by a combination of bacteria, sebum, and dead skin cells. The clogs occur deep within the skin and are further below the surface than nodules.

These large red or white bumps are often painful to the touch. Cysts are the largest form of acne, and their formation usually results from a severe infection. This type of acne is also the most likely to scar.

The prescription medication isotretinoin (Sotret) is commonly used to treat cysts. In severe cases, your dermatologist may surgically remove a cyst.

Types

67

Stress can be a key trigger of acne in some cases.

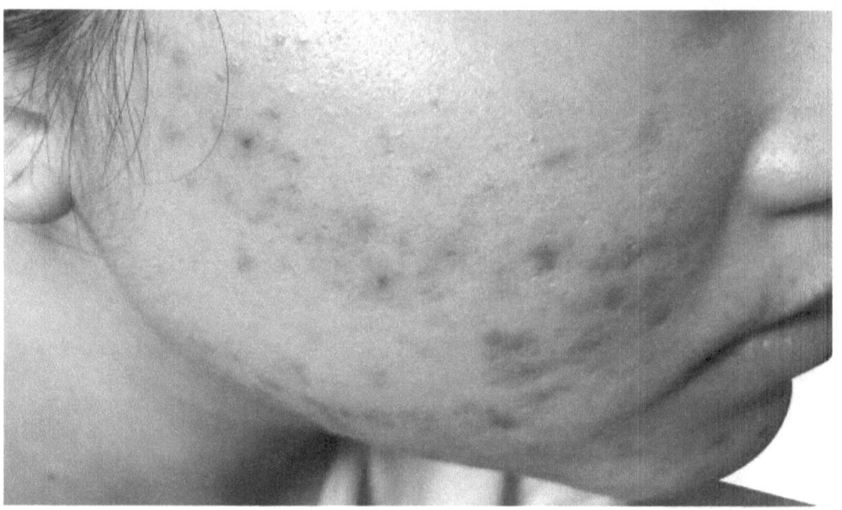

Acne pimples vary in size, color, and level of pain.

The following types are possible:

Whiteheads: These remain under the skin and are small

Blackheads: Clearly visible, they are black and appear on the surface of the skin

Papules: Small, usually pink bumps, these are visible on the surface of the skin

Pustules: Clearly visible on the surface of the skin.

They are red at their base and have pus at the top

Nodules: Clearly visible on the surface of the skin. They are large, solid, painful pimples that are embedded deep in the skin

69

Cysts: Clearly visible on the surface of the skin. They are painful and filled with pus. Cysts can cause scars.

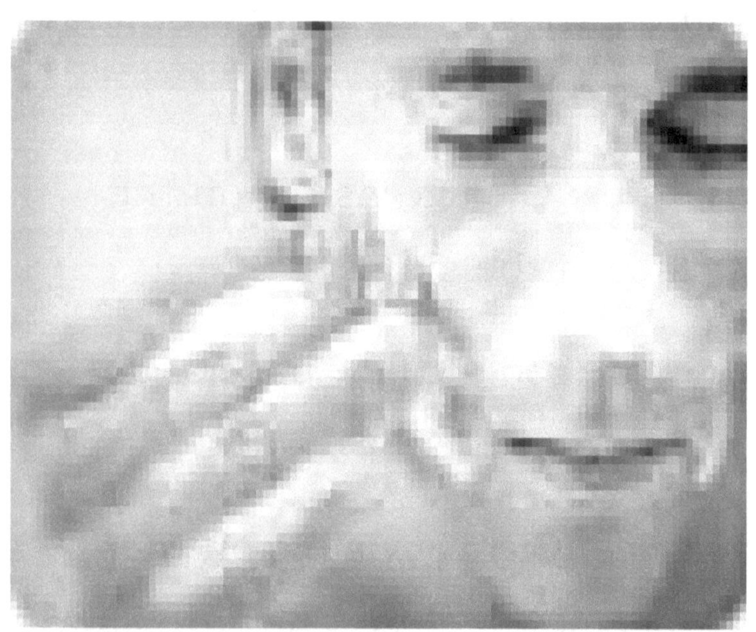

Prevention and management tips

Here are some tips for looking after skin that has acne or is prone to it.

- Wash your face no more than twice each day with warm water and mild soap made especially for acne.

- Do not scrub the skin or burst the pimples, as this may push the infection further down, causing more blocking, swelling, and redness.

- Avoid popping pimples, as this makes scarring likelier.

71

- A specialist can treat a pimple that requires rapid removal for cosmetic reasons.

- Refrain from touching the face.

- Hold the telephone away from the face when talking, as it is likely to contain sebum and skin residue.

- Wash hands frequently, especially before applying lotions, creams, or makeup.

- Clean spectacles regularly as they collect sebum and skin residue.

- If acne is on the back, shoulders, or chest, try wearing

loose clothing to let the skin breathe.

- Avoid tight garments, such as headbands, caps, and scarves, or wash them regularly if used.

- Choose makeup for sensitive skin and avoid oil-based products. Remove makeup before sleeping.

- Use an electric shaver or sharp safety razors when shaving.

- Soften the skin and beard with warm soapy water before applying shaving cream.

- Keep hair clean, as it collects sebum and skin residue. Avoid greasy hair products, such as those containing cocoa butter.

- Avoid excessive sun exposure, as it can cause the skin to produce more sebum. Several acne medications increase the risk of <u>sunburn</u>.

- Avoid anxiety and stress, as it can increase production of cortisol and adrenaline, which exacerbate acne.

- Try to keep cool and dry in hot and humid climates, to prevent sweating. Acne is a common problem. It can cause severe embarrassment, but treatment is available, and it is effective in many cases.

Other Book from the same Author

https://www.amazon.com/dp/B0822XLQXD

Related Topics

Acne be gone for good, acne diet, Acne rx, Acne scars, Acne mask, Acne Skin Products, Ace atkins, acne no you can heal your life, Acne patches, healing back pain, heal your body, eat to beat disease, rosemary gladstar's medicinal herbs, how to starve cancer, acne treatment, red light therapy, healing psoriasis, the eczema diet, milady standard esthetics,

76

acne wipes, acne xl patch more, acne scars, acne treatment, acne skin products, Acne mask, acne dermatology, Acne dots, acne mask, acne dots, the hidden cause of acne, getting clear, the beauty of dirty skin, the clear skin diet, acne cure, the alpha skin care essential renewal lotion | anti aging formula, real solutions for adult acne, the skin care answer, clean skin from within, medical medium liver rescue, medical medium celery juice, medical medium life changing foods, medical medium, medical medium thyroid healing, hidden healing powers of super whole foods, summary analysis of medical medium liver rescue, summary of medical medium liver rescue by Anthony William, natural liver flush, skinny liver, the teachings of acne, put your best face forward, the acne prescription, the beauty geek's guide to skin care puritans pride zinc for acne 100 count, Â¿cÃ³mo curar el acnÃ© [how to cure acne], quit acne, skin cleanse, quit pms, the acne answer, what your acne is trying to tell you, the hormonal acne solution, dirty looks , understanding skin flip chart, younger skin starts in the gut, the skincare bible, acne face mask, anne graham lotz.

Content Credits:

https://www.webmd.com/skin-problems-and-treatments/acne/picture-of-acne

https://www.aad.org/diseases/acne/acne-overview

Images Sources

Getty images

Feedback Reviews

We have finally come to the end of this eBook.

If you enjoyed this book

And learnt from it too,

Why not then go online

To write a Sweet review!

Just a line of Phrase will be fine.

Thank you so much.....................